Michel
Montignac

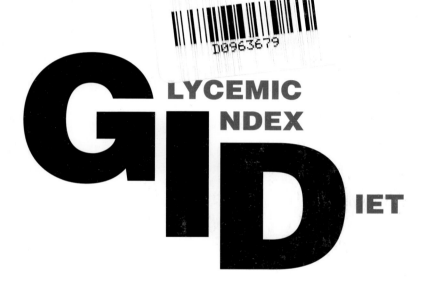

D0963679

GLYCEMIC INDEX DIET

for Weight Loss

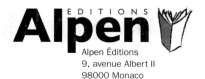

EDITIONS
Alpen

Alpen Éditions
9, avenue Albert II
98000 Monaco

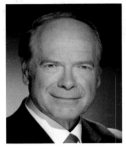

In 1986 Michel Montignac was the first person in the world to introduce glycemic index as a weight loss concept. Today he is still a world expert in applying this concept to prevent and reduce weight gain and obesity.

Official website: **www.montignac.com**

Shop online: **www.montignac-shop.com**

Coaching online: **www.methode-montignac.com**

Exclusive copyrights:
©Alpen Éditions
9, avenue Albert II
98000 Monaco
Tel: +377 97 77 62 10
Fax: +377 97 77 62 11
web: www.alpen.mc

Printed in Italy
ISBN: 978-2-35934-037-2

Michel
Montignac

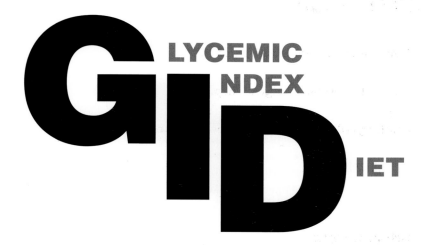

GLYCEMIC **I**NDEX **D**IET

for Weight Loss

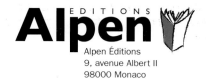

EDITIONS
Alpen

Alpen Éditions
9, avenue Albert II
98000 Monaco

CONTENTS

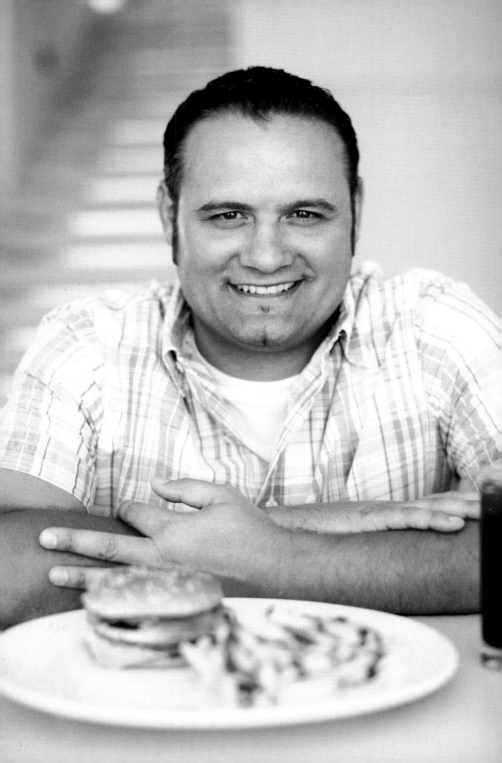

Introduction

Obesity levels increased considerably in the last century, to the extent that the World Health Organization (WHO) declared it to be a true epidemic in 1997. Figure 1 shows the increases.

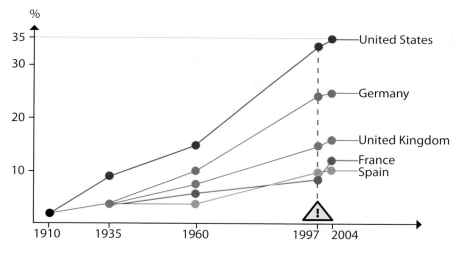

Figure 1. **Obesity Rates in the 20th Century**

What we need to remember is that for a little over 50 years the official solution suggested for stamping out excessive weight gain was based upon this hypothesis: *"If you are fat, it's because you eat too much and you don't exercise enough."*

The recommendation that flowed from that was that we have to eat fewer calories, and in particular less fat, because fat contains many calories, and especially that we should do much more exercise. This meant diets prescribed by practitioners were low-calorie, and most doctors and nutritionists still use those today.

The best known nutritionists, whether in France where I am or elsewhere, still recommend 1,200 calorie-per-day, low-fat, crash diets to overweight people.

We should recognize that this type of diet, often widely practiced, as is the case in the United States, for example, has absolutely not managed to curb rising obesity for 50 years, not only in western countries, but also in developing countries and in particular in eastern Europe, the Middle East and Asia.

This is why, since 1960, many epidemiological studies have been undertaken in western countries to try to show any correlation between obesity rates in developed societies and a number of environmental factors. The results of these studies were so unexpected and surprising that they were called the "**nutritional paradox.**"

According to these epidemiological studies, average daily calorie consumption in western countries dropped by about 35% over the last 50 years. During the same period, obesity increased by more than 400% in the USA and more than 300% in Europe. Let's use French statistics as an example.

Figure 2 below shows, for example, that the change is particularly significant in France.

	1935	1960	2003	↘ since 1935	↘ since 1960
MEN	3 100	2 800	**2 196**	41 %	27,5 %
WOMEN	2 500	2 300	**1 570**	59 %	46 %
Total population change				↘ 50 %	↘ 36 %

Figure 2. **Comparison between French calorie intake in 2003, 1960, and 1935.**

According to various studies (OBépi 2003, Suvimax 2003), French daily calorie consumption dropped between 1960 and 2003 by:

- 27.5% for men, and

- 46% for women

This is an average reduction of **36%** for the whole French population.

Yet as we saw before, obesity increased threefold in France in the same period.

We also see from the same Figure that calorie intake in France has dropped by 50% since 1935. This means that we eat half as much as our grandparents did in the first half of the 20th century. In France it is not hard to believe this, when we look at the menus for banquets celebrating baptisms, communions, and weddings of that era.

It is interesting to note in Figure 3 that, according to the last Suvimax study in 2003, the French are said to eat 20% less than nutritionists' official recommendations. But they keep on getting fatter!

	Official recommendations 1980 (kcal/d)	SUVIMAX reality 2003	Gap
MEN	2 500	2 196	-14 %
WOMEN	2 000	1 570	-27 %
		Average:	-20 %

Figure 3. The difference between daily calorie intake in France and official recommendations.

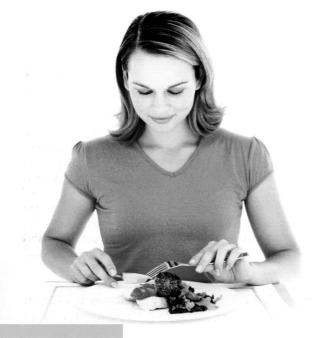

The Suvimax study, performed on 13,000 representative French people during the period 1995-2003, also shows us that the French:

- eat less fat

- eat more carbohydrates

- eat the same amount of protein

- spend more time exercising.

In conclusion, the study shows that French calorie intake over the period (8 years) dropped by 6%, and that paradoxically, over the same period obesity increased by 31%.

Other statistical studies show that the time the French spend exercising has doubled in the 40 years. In English-speaking countries, where the prevalence of obesity is much higher than in France, time spent exercising has increased by even higher proportions.

There are other paradoxes in the results of these epidemiological studies. For example, it is in the socioeconomic categories where most exercise is done during working hours that most obesity is found.

This is the case for agricultural workers, tradesmen, or cleaning ladies, for example. Conversely, sedentary people (managers in particular) are least obese.

Another paradox: in countries where fat consumption is lowest overall (lower than official recommendations), obesity is highest. In South Africa, for example, fat represents 22% of daily calorie intake (rather than the 30% recommended by nutritionists) whereas average Body Mass Index (BMI), which measures the prevalence of obesity, is 59 as compared to an ideal of 25. The same is the case for Saudi Arabia, where fat consumption is 24% but the BMI is 49. Paradoxically, Cretans, who eat 45% fat as compared to the 30% recommended, have a Body Mass Index of 24, lower than the ideal of 25.

So from these scientific studies we see that in contrast to what we have long believed, <u>there is no correlation between the corpulence of a population and its calorie intake</u>. There is no correlation with the level of exercise either. Therefore, we conclude that we have been wrong in thinking that the energy factor was a determining factor in weight gain. The calories in our food are obviously not entirely unrelated to weight gain, but we must admit that this is a secondary factor. We also know from statistics analyzed by Professor Creff on thousands of obese patients that only 15% of obese people eat excessively.

Today we know that because of a person's digestive physiology and how metabolism occurs that other, more complex factors are at play in how we gain weight, and even more so in how we become obese. We know that intestinal absorption modulates nutrient bioavailability, and we also know that a meal's energy (in terms of calories) is either burned or stored as fat, as a function of metabolic processes caused by the **nature** of the food.

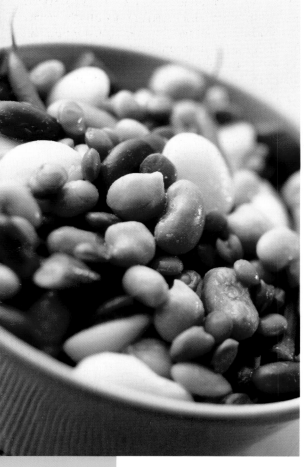

In fact, whether the metabolic process orients the meal's energy toward storage or toward burning (and vice versa) depends on the **nature** of the food consumed.

The **nature** of the food depends on a number of factors:

- the physical and chemical structure (for example the type of starch for a carbohydrate, the type of fatty acid for a fat, the type of protein);

- any fiber they contain; the type of fiber; whether it is soluble or not;

- the protein content and where this protein comes from;

- how the food is physically treated (whether it is raw or cooked, and the temperature at which it is cooked).

These factors mean that for two identical foods, the absorption level can be completely different, and therefore, set off divergent metabolic reactions leading to either the meal's energy being burned, or to the fat being stored, thus to weight gain. An example would be portions with the same number of calories of two complex carbohydrates such as potatoes on one hand and lentils on the other.

To better understand how the various metabolic scenarios can lead to either weight gain or to weight loss two essential metabolic ideas must be understood: glycemia and insulin secretion.

Glycemia

Glycemia is the amount of sugar (glucose, in fact) in the blood.

After fasting, in the morning, glycemia levels are about 1 gram per liter of blood. When we eat a carbohydrate (at breakfast for example), it is transformed into glucose during digestion. This extra glucose then appears in the blood, increasing glycemia until it reaches a peak.

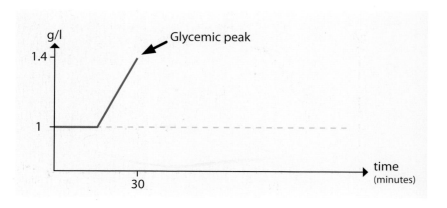

Figure 4. **Reaching the glycemic peak after eating a carbohydrate**

Insulin secretion

The pancreas then secretes a hormone, insulin, to remove the glucose from the blood and store it in muscle tissue and the liver (glycogen).

The insulin response reduces glycemia, so in theory the glycemia curve then drops again to its baseline level.

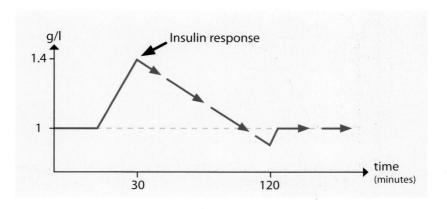

Figure 5. **Insulin response**

The Insulin Response

Consider two cases: one for slim people and one for overweight people.

• In a slim person, the amount of insulin secreted is exactly proportional to the glycemia level. The pancreas will therefore secrete exactly the insulin dose required to reduce glycemia. When the glycemia has returned to its baseline, there is no more insulin (figure 6).

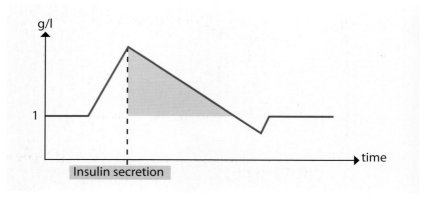

Figure 6. **In a slim person the insulin response is proportional to glycemia.**

• In an overweight person more insulin will be secreted than is needed to reduce glycemia. At the end of the process, when glycemia has dropped, there will be **residual insulin** that we call **hyperinsulinism**. (Figure 7)

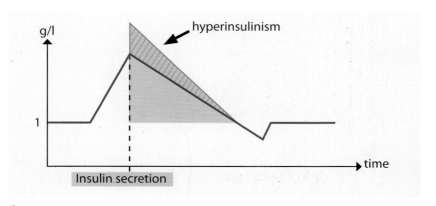

Figure 7. **In an overweight person, the insulin response is disproportionate. This residual insulin is hyperinsulinism.**

Hyperinsulinism: the cause of weight gain

When insulin secretion is <u>normal</u>, most of a meal's energy is burned using the following processes:

- **lipogenesis** (fat storage) is inhibited,

- **lipolysis** (use of fat stores) is stimulated by activation of a special enzyme, **triglyceride lipase**.

Conversely, when insulin secretion is <u>disproportionate</u> (residual insulin) part of the meal's energy is stored as fat, because of these processes:

- **lipogenesis** is stimulated by the activation of another enzyme, **lipoprotein lipase** by insulin.

- **lipolysis** is inhibited.

In other words if there is residual insulin after the meal is digested, weight can be gained; this is why we state that <u>hyperinsulinism is the cause of weight gain</u>, and that all those who have a weight problem have hyperinsulinemia to varying degrees. This is also how we discover that to trigger weight loss, we have to <u>reduce</u> glycemia, to reduce the <u>insulin response</u>.

Two comparable carbohydrates can cause different glycemia

To better understand these phenomena we can do the following little experiment. Let's examine the relative metabolic effects of eating two comparable foods: **potatoes** on one hand and **lentils** on the other. These two foods can be compared because they belong to the same food group, carbohydrates, and more specifically they are both starches, i.e. complex carbohydrates. For the comparison to be significant, the portions have to have the same number of calories, let's say 400 kcal.

After having eaten the portion of potatoes, we see that about 80% of the starch that it contains has been transformed into glucose by digestive amylases, and this glucose, after having crossed the stomach wall, is seen in a **high** rise in **glycemia**.

In contrast, after having eaten the same portion calorie-wise of lentils we see that only about 20% of the starch that they contain is transformed into glucose by digestive enzymes. This means very **low glycemia**. The legitimate question that we should ask is why eating potatoes causes high glycemia, whereas eating the same portion calorie-wise of lentils causes much lower (four times lower) glycemia.

What makes the glycemia difference is the **nature** of the respective **starches**.
Potato starch is **soft** and composed largely of amylopectin, which is easily transformed into glucose by digestive amylases. The starch in lentils is different: it is **strong**, because it is made mainly of amylose and cannot easily be transformed into glucose by digestive enzymes.

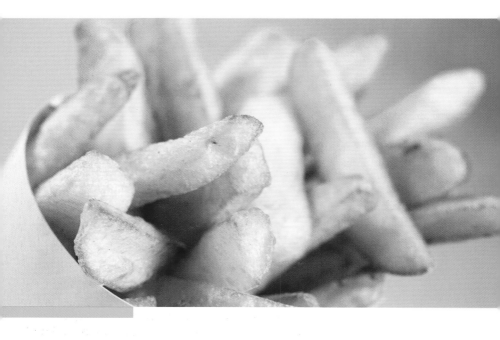

Metabolic effects

Let us now look at the metabolic effects in each example and the consequences of different glycemia levels. We want to evaluate the metabolic effects induced. With potatoes, glycemia is high so there is a high insulin response; lipogenesis (and lipolysis inhibition) are activated. Consequently there is a risk of <u>fat being stored</u> instead of burned. There are also side effects.

There is a risk of <u>hypoglycemia</u> (because the higher the postprandial insulin the greater the glycemia drop, to the point where it can fall below the norm (1 g/l).

This gives specific symptoms:

- fatigue, which is the well-known after-meal fatigue,

- hunger, so there is a strong desire to snack.

With lentils, we have seen that glycemic incidence was low. The metabolic effect will therefore be different. Only a low insulin effect will be seen, which means lipogenesis inhibition and lipolysis activation. So there will be <u>no risk of storage</u>, and the meal's energy will be <u>burned</u>.

And what about side effects?

Since <u>glycemia is low</u>, there is no risk of hypoglycemia, which means there is no notable fatigue, a good feeling of satiety, and no need to snack.

<u>We can therefore conclude</u> that two comparable carbohydrates can have different, even opposite metabolic reactions. This is precisely what <u>glycemic index</u> measures.

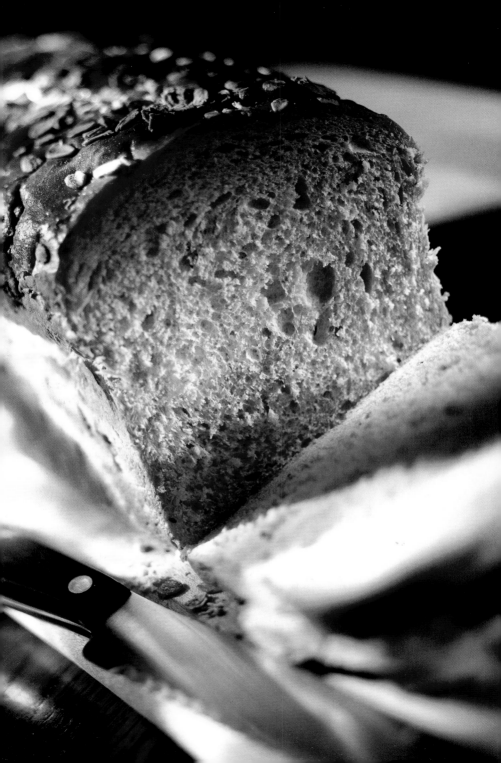

Glycemic Index

Glycemic index measures the ability of a carbohydrate (for equal pure carbohydrate content) to raise glycemia compared to a scale of values built by taking pure glucose as a reference.

All carbohydrates have been placed on the glycemic index scale based upon their <u>nature</u> or <u>how they are metabolized</u>.

Discovering Glycemic Index

For a long time, we considered that all carbohydrates were equal at equal amounts, and had the same effect on glycemia. This is why when doctors discovered one of their patients was diabetic, they recommended that the patient stop eating carbohydrates (fruit, cereals, pulses, etc.). This was restrictive diet that was almost impossible to follow.

Thankfully, in the mid 1970s, a researcher at the University of Stanford in the USA (P.A. Crapo) showed just the opposite through various experiments, i.e. that carbohydrates had differing effects on glycemia. So Crapo was the first to show through several studies that diabetics could continue to eat carbohydrates as long as they had a low effect on glycemia. These experiments showed that diabetes could be stabilized, or even reduced, by simply selecting carbohydrates carefully.

In 1981, a researcher at the University of Toronto in Canada, David Jenkins, continuing the work of Crapo, developed a hierarchy of carbohydrates based upon their effect on glycemia. He gave each of them an index, calculated compared to pure glucose, which was given the value of 100. The index of 100 given arbitrarily to glucose represented the surface area of the area under the corresponding hyperglycemia curve. From this, the glycemic index of the other carbohydrates, for a given quantity of pure carbohydrate (50 g) is calculated using the following formula:

$$\frac{Surface\ area\ under\ the\ curve\ for\ the\ carbohydrate\ tested}{Surface\ area\ under\ the\ curve\ for\ glucose} \times 100$$

The glycemic index therefore is higher or lower in relation to the hyperglycemia caused (see figure 8).

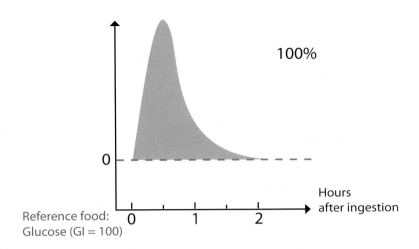

100%

Hours
after ingestion

Reference food:
Glucose (GI = 100)

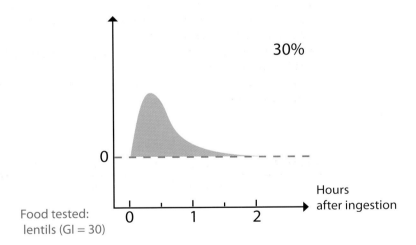

30%

Hours
after ingestion

Food tested:
lentils (GI = 30)

Figure 8: **Glycemia curve two hours after ingesting first glucose then lentils with identical amounts of carbohydrate (50 g)**

Crapo and Jenkins were diabetes specialists. They worked on the variation in carbohydrates' effect on glycemia and development of the table of glycemic indexes to give diabetics more comfortable nutritional options, but it was especially done to add a new concept diabetes treatment by encouraging disease specialists to adjust their therapies as a consequence. So the least we can say is that this discovery, at the time, did not raise much enthusiasm in the little closeted world of diabetology where, just like many areas of medicine, people are very careful of revolutionary ideas.

Thus the concept of glycemic index stayed embryonic after it was first developed, and still today more than 25 years later, it is often treated with indifference by diabetes specialists, in spite of all the studies that have been published since then on its therapeutic value.

The "Fast Sugar" and "Slow Sugar" Classification is False!

For a long time, nutritionists have classified carbohydrates in two quite distinct categories, according to how long it takes for them to be assimilated by the body. The categories are "fast sugars" and "slow sugars".

Under "fast sugars" (more specifically, fast carbohydrates) were single sugars and double sugars such as glucose and saccharose, which are contained in particular in sugar cane and sugar beet. These names were based on the belief that they were assimilated rapidly, shortly after ingestion, because of the simplicity of their carbohydrate molecule.

Conversely, the "slow sugar" category (i.e. slow carbohydrates) contained all the carbohydrates whose molecules are complex (starches) where we thought that glucose release happened slowly and progressively in the body because of the more complex chemical transformation necessary. This is why fruits were "fast sugars" (digested quickly) whereas potatoes and bread were "slow sugars" (digested slowly).

In 1978 Australian scientist M. L. Wahlqvist demonstrated that this belief was completely wrong. His experiments proved that "the complexity of the carbohydrate molecule does not affect the rate at which the glucose is released and assimilated by the body."

We see that the glycemic peak for all carbohydrates (i.e. the maximum absorption), regardless of whether they are simple or complex and taken in isolation after fasting, takes the same time (about half an hour after ingestion). The rate of carbohydrate assimilation is not therefore specific, from one carbohydrate to another, as we have thought for a long time. From this we see that carbohydrates should be studied as a function of the glycemia that they cause. This is precisely what the concept of glycemic index does, as we have already discussed.

The Controversial Years

Personally I discovered the concept of glycemic index in 1980 when I was working in the USA for a multinational pharmaceutical company. I had always been obsessed about being overweight. I had been an obese child, and was in a never-ending search for information that might help me solve my weight problem forever. I took advantage of working in a scientific environment to perfect documentation on this subject that was so important to me.

Although they only involved diabetes, Crapo's 1976 studies intrigued me. More than 85% of diabetics are also obese, so it was not an unreasonable hypothesis that the diet developed for diabetics might have beneficial effects on all obese people. In any case, I wouldn't lose anything by seeing whether it did.

This is how I lost 16 kilos in three months during my time in the US, then five more kilos in the months that followed by following, let us remember, a diet for diabetics, and I wasn't a diabetic.

I had shown that choosing between what, at that time, I called "good" and "bad" carbohydrates at the time was an effective means of losing weight, while continuing to eat normally without any calorie restrictions. The basic principle of the Montignac Method, which it would become after publication of my first book in 1986, was therefore set.

The immediate success of this first book, which was targeted specifically to business men, and especially of the second book (*"Je mange donc je maigris* [I Eat, Therefore I Lose Weight]") published in 1987 for the mass market, led to immediate criticism from nutritionists and other dieticians who believed that all carbohydrates were good for us. After having dragged me through the mud and calling me an imposter and a quack, they gave me a chance to explain myself in more scientific terms.

In the subsequent editions of my books I tried to justify my classification of "good" and "bad" carbohydrates by further developing the concept of glycemic index. The criticism only became more scathing, and they called me a sorcerer's apprentice. The more famous professors even shouted from the rooftops to decry my deceit in a long article with the evocative title *"Pour en finir avec la méthode Montignac !* [Enough of the Montignac Method!]" published in *"Quotidien du médecin* [Doctor's Daily]" on October 7, 1993. This article said it was dangerous to talk to the public about *"ideas unknown in the medical world, unvalidated in their own field, diabetology, that have absolutely nothing to do with weight gain."* Doctor Fricker, who was at the front of the anti-Montignac line, concluded then, and for many years after, that *"the Montignac diet* [based upon glycemic indexes] *was an intellectual con and dangerous to health."* As only fools never change their minds, we should pay homage to the same Dr. Fricker today, as his latest weight-loss books recommend that people should not eat potatoes or white bread because of their high glycemic index!

Until the end of the 1990's the concept of glycemic index was not only given the cold shoulder, it was violently attacked by nutrition professionals. And the Montignac Method, which had been the first to use GI as its foundational principle, was not only ridiculed and castigated, but systematically denounced by its detractors.

However, thankfully, this did not stop its effective development by virtue of word of mouth, in France and abroad where more than 18 million books on the Montignac Method have been sold since the first publication.

Long-Overdue Recognition

In 1997, the Food and Agriculture Organization (FAO) and the World Health Organization (WHO), two important UN bodies, denounced the endemic prevalence of world obesity and officially recognized that the concept of glycemic index could be of help in fighting this scourge.

It should be said that by the end of the 20th century, a number of diabetology researchers who had not really been convinced of the value of glycemic indexes in their own domain had been more successful by demonstrating how useful it is in preventing weight gain. These studies were mainly epidemiological studies though, published in particular under the responsibility of Professor Walter Willette at the School of Public Health at Harvard in the USA. He established undeniable correlations between obesity and excessive consumption of low glycemic index carbohydrates, and conversely between consumption of low glycemic index carbohydrates and prevention of weight loss.

For ten years, a large number of scientific studies have directly or indirectly demonstrated the value of glycemic index in fighting obesity and also in preventing diabetes and cardiovascular disease. All this is really wonderful validation of the Montignac Method, which was the first in the world, more than 20 years ago, to suggest using the concept of glycemic index for weight loss.

Unfortunately, this concept has become a fashion of some sort in recent years, with many general practitioners and even journalists who have no right to be writing on this subject, feeling they were able to talk about their pseudo-understanding by publishing books for the mass market on glycemic index, when they had neither the experience, nor the expertise. So in wanting to popularize knowledge over which they did not have mastery, these ignoramuses often compromised credibility by over-working the principles.

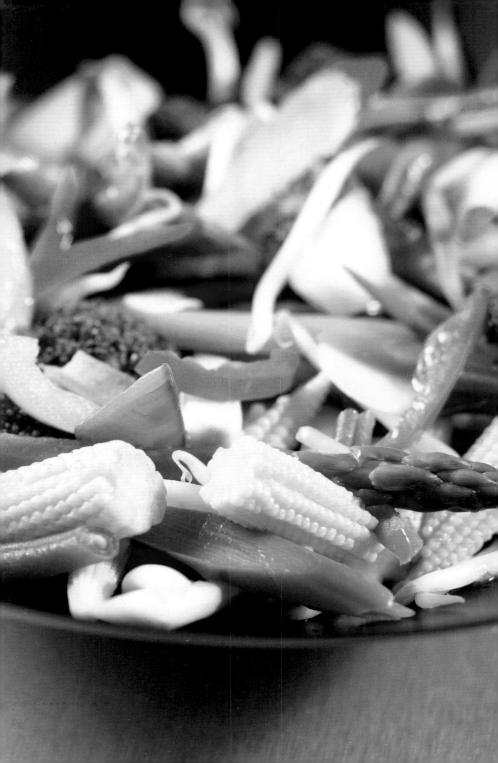

Analyzing the GI table

As we have already seen, glycemic index measures how a carbohydrate raises glycemia (blood sugar) after being ingested and more specifically digested.

The glycemic index table was created using glucose, the purest carbohydrate, as a reference with a value of 100. Opposite you will see a simplified table in which the most common foods appear. There is a more complete table in the second section of the book.

In this chapter the focus is on analyzing the distribution of foods that we have so-far classified into two columns: On the left carbohydrates with high glycemic indexes (from 55 to 100), and on the right, carbohydrates with low (from 40 to 50) and very low glycemic indexes (from 0 to 35).

Table of Glycemic Indexes (GI)

High GI carbohydrates		Low and Very-low GI carbohydrates	
Maltose (beer)	110	Brown rice	50
Glucose	100	Long-grain basmati rice	50
Modified starch	100	Sweet potato	50
Baked potatoes	95	Whole-wheat pasta	50
Fried potatoes	95	Sugar-free, whole grain cereals/muesli	45
Rice flour	95	
White hamburger buns	85	Whole grain rye bread	45
Cooked carrots	85	Standard whole wheat bread	45/50
Corn flakes, pop corn	85	Pumpernickel bread	40
Instant/parboiled rice	85	Porridge oats	40
Rice pudding	85	Kidney beans	40
Puffed rice (Rice Crispies)	85	Fresh fruit juice (no added sugar)	40
Mashed potato	80	Spaghetti al dente (5 min)	40
Cooked broad beans	80	Long grain Montignac brown basmati rice	40
Pumpkin, watermelon	75	
Sugar (saccharose)	70	Whole what pasta *al dente*	35
White bread (e.g. baguettes)	70	Figs, dried apricots, prunes	35
Refined sweetened cereals	70	Indian corn	35
Chocolate bars	70	Fresh peas	35
Boiled, peeled potatoes	70	Wild rice	35
		Quinoa	35
Potato chips	70	Montignac whole wheat bread	34

High GI carbohydrates		Low and Very-low GI carbohydrates	
Soda	70	Raw carrots, tomatoes	30
Cookies	70	Dairy products	30
White rice	70	Dried white beans	30
Pasta, ravioli	70	Lentils (brown or yellow)	30
Sweet corn	65	Chick peas	30
Raisins	65	Other fresh fruit (apples, pears, oranges, apricots, etc.)	30
Partially whole grain bread	65		
Boiled, unpeeled potatoes	65	Green beans	30
		Soy noodles	30
Beet	65	Montignac sugar-free marmalade	25
Whole-weat bread	65	Green lentils	25
Standard sweetened jams	60/65	Flageolet beans	25
Honey	60	Split peas	25
Refined semolina/couscous	60	Dark chocolate (> 70% cacao)	25
Long-grain white rice	60	Garlic, onions	20
Ripe bananas	55	Montignac fructose	20
Melon	55	Green vegetables, green beans, lettuce	15
Well-cooked white spaghetti	55		
Shortbread	55	Eggplant	15
		Soy beans (edamame)	15
		Peanuts, walnuts, hazelnuts, almonds	15

More complete tables are given in the second part of the book

In the left-hand column, there are mainly modern and industrially processed foods.

Foods with high GI that are in the left-hand column are usually modern foods that have only been eaten for less than two centuries.

- **Sugar**

Before the early 19th century sugar was hardly ever present in everyday cooking. It was extracted only from sugar cane produced in the New World. Therefore it was very expensive and could only be purchased from apothecaries.

In 1800, sugar consumption in Europe was less than 1 kg per person, per year. After the process of extracting sugar from beet was developed in 1812 the product became common and its consumption increased exponentially (see the table for statistics)

	France	Other countries (2005)
1800	0,6 kg	UK : 35 kg
1880	8 kg	Spain : 32 kg
1900	17 kg	Italy : 30 kg
1930	30 kg	USA : 63 kg[*]
1965	40 kg	Australia : 46 kg
1990	35 kg	Japan : 19 kg
2005	33 kg	China : 8 kg

* This is a little more than 50% of sugar equivalents, because Americans essentially eat glucose that has come from corn.

**History of sugar consumption in France
and current consumption in other countries**
(Number of kg per year, per person)

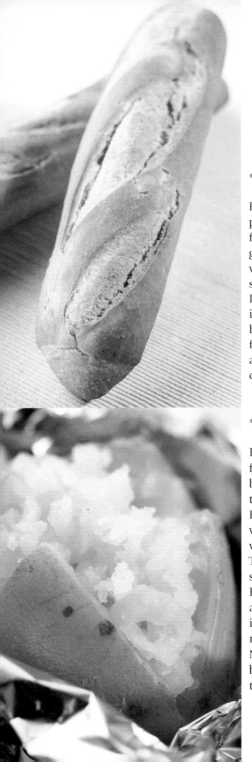

- **Refined flour**

For centuries bread eaten by most of the population was made with crude milled flours (whole grains) or partially whole grain flour (bolted flour). White flower was rare and expensive because it was sifted by hand.

It took till 1870 when the roll mill was invented for most of the population to have access to refined flour, called white flour, which became whiter and whiter after the Second World War so that it could be stored for longer.

- **Potatoes**

Potatoes did not exist in the common food of most countries either at the beginning of the 19th century. For a long time they had been used to fatten pigs. In France for example, during the revolution when famine became a threat, potatoes were introduced into the human diet. They have been eaten more and more since that time.

From the table we see that when potatoes are boiled in their skins their glycemic index is average (65). This used to be the most common method of preparing them. Nowadays potatoes are most often eaten baked or fried, and GI values for these types of potatoes are very high (95).

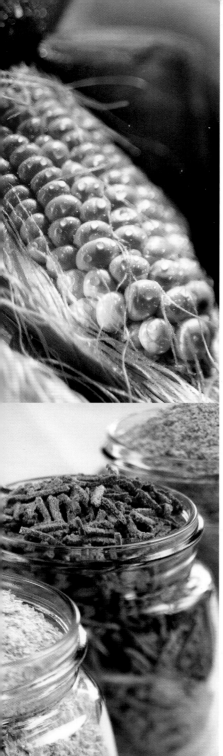

- **Hybrid and genetically modified cereals**

These cereals also have high GI and are in the table's left-hand column. In particular, we are talking about modern sweet corn whose GI is 70.

Corn was discovered when America was. It was the staple food of Native Americans and its GI was very low (35). Since it gave low yields, botanists have been trying to make a more productive plant ever since.

Modern sweet corn is the result of a long series of hybridizations and other genetic modifications that have improved corn's yield considerably but with the side effect of a large rise in glycemic index. This is the price we have paid.

- **Synthesized foods, and industrially processed foods**

These foods are also in the table of high GI. These are largely preservatives, gellants, modified starches, starches and the like whose GI approach 100.

We should note that extruded, popped or puffed cereals like corn flakes, pop corn and puffed rice have higher GI than the unprocessed cereal.

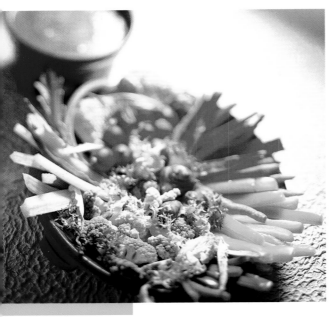

In the right-hand column, most of the foods were eaten by our ancestors

In particular we find natural foods there:

- unrefined complete cereals, in particular old-fashioned bread (whole-grain bread) ,

- ancient grains: buckwheat, rye, spelt, kamut, quinoa, etc.

- pasta made with durum wheat

- ancient, unhybridized rice like basmati

- fruit

- vegetables

- legumes and pulses, which are eaten ten times less than they were a century ago : lentils, beans, peas, chick peas (garbanzo beans), and soy, which we have discovered from Asian cuisine.

These foods are essentially what our parents, grandparents and great-grandparents used to eat, and it is why being overweight was three to four times less likely then than now in western populations

It is easy to understand why more than a third of Americans are obese.

When we look at the typical diet we see why Americans have the world's highest obesity rates.

It is because the essential features of the American dietary model are high GI carbohydrates:

- Sugar (63 kg/year/person, i.e. twice as much as Europeans)

- Refined flours are the basis of hamburger and hot dog buns, pizzas, cookies, crackers, and chips.

- Sweet corn from hybrids whose GI is 70 is consumed daily in other forms like corn flakes or pop corn whose GI is even higher (85).

- Industrially processed foods represent 3/4 of the foods eaten in the US.

- Fried potatoes and potato chips, which are eaten at all meals, even sometimes for breakfast (e.g. hash browns).

So Americans eat a diet containing much high GI food that is hyperglycemiant, and therefore hyperinsulinemiant, which (as we have already seen) leads to hypoglycemia and systematically to snacking. The consequence is general weight gain and eventually obesity!

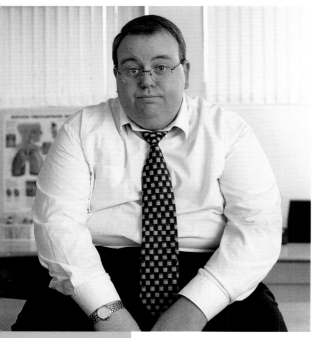

Why are people in parts of Europe slimmer?

In Latinate countries (France, Spain, Italy, Portugal, Greece) obesity is two times lower than in the United States and much lower than in English-speaking countries in general.

For essentially cultural reasons, populations of Latinate origin have kept traditional eating habits that mean spending longer in preparing meals from fresh ingredients and in general in eating many more low-GI foods (e.g. fruit, vegetables, and legumes).

In spite of the way the modern socio-professional life is organized, people in these countries eat three times less processed food than Americans (they cook more), eat half as much sugar and refined cereals and consequently they snack much less. Therefore we can deduce that the average glycemic index for a country's eating habits predicts its population's obesity level!

Drifting eating habits

We ought to consider that the worldwide obesity epidemic that the WHO decreed is the result of a slow drift in eating habits that began in the early 20th century, with more and more high-GI carbohydrates and fewer and fewer low-GI carbohydrates being eaten.

The main reason for this drift, which leads to increased obesity everywhere it occurs, is without doubt the adoption of the North American way of eating. Its symbols are hamburgers and Coca Cola.

Globalization of eating habits means unfortunately that this American-style diet is taking root in other places. Our conclusion is that glycemic index is a crucial criterion in preventing weight gain, and for weight loss, as many scientific studies have shown.

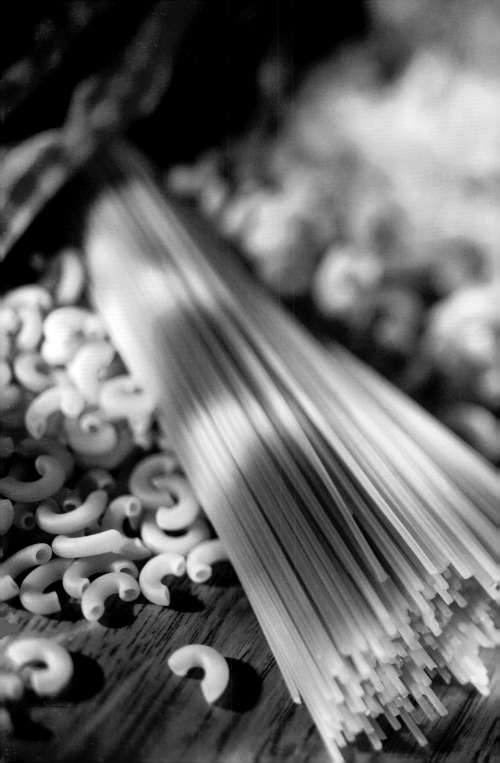

Factors that modify Glycemic Index

Most carbohydrates commonly eaten by humans are complex, composed essentially of starch.

Therefore they are part of the category of foods called amylaceous foods, which can itself be split into four categories (cf p53).

To be absorbed into the blood system all of these starches have to be transformed into glucose. It is digestive enzymes (alpha amylases in particular) that do this work.

Digestion begins in the mouth with chewing, and continues in the small intestine after passing through the stomach.

Rising glycemia shows when the glucose has been absorbed and therefore how digestible a particular starch is. The size of the rise is measure by the glycemic index scale, as we have seen in the preceding chapters. The observation was that for a given amount of carbohydrate, from one food to another, postprandial glycemia level could vary widely, because there is some starch that resists digestion, so there is varying absorption.

Several factors cause this variation in starch digestibility, which is still measured by glycemic index.

Starch's structure:

A grain of starch is composed of two types of molecular components: **amylose and amylopectin**. They can be combined with lipids, proteins, fiber and micronutrients (vitamins, minerals, etc.). It is essentially the proportion of amylose in comparison with amylopectin that determines the physicochemical nature of amylaceous foods and how they are metabolized in humans.

Cereals	Tubers	Legumes	Fruits
Common wheat	Potatoes	Beans of all kinds	Bananas
Durum wheat	Sweet potatoes	Peas	Mangos
Rice	Manioc	Chick peas	Apples
Corn	Yam	Lentils	
Oats	Taro		
Barley	Tania		
Rye			
Sorghum			
Millet			

Amylaceous families

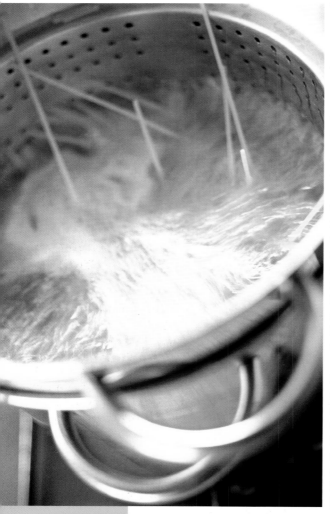

This amylose/amylopectin ratio can vary widely from one botanical family to another and from one variety to another within a given family.

Starches in cereal generally contain between 15-28% amylose, but there are varieties of corn that contain less than 1%, like the waxy corns whose extracts are used in the food industry as thickeners. In contrast, other varieties of corn contain 55-80% but are not commonly cultivated, because the higher the amylose content, the lower the yield. This was the case for Indian corn.

Starches from tubers have much lower amylose content (from 17- 22%). e.g. potatoes. Starches from legumes such as lentils, beans, and chick peas have much higher amylose content (33-66%).

Variations in glycemic index

The glycemic index of an amylaceous food varies according to a number of parameters:

- **The amylose-amylopectin ratio**

Since amylose is a starch that resists amylase digestion, for any food the higher the amylose content, the lower its glycemic index and vice versa.

- **Heating and moisture retention**

When heated in excess water, starch's structure changes. Grains of starch swell progressively and a fraction of amylopectin dissolves. If heating is for an extended period a fraction of amylose also dissolves.

The result is that the viscosities of the suspensions vary. This phenomenon is called starch <u>gelatinization</u>.

The lower the proportion of amylose, the higher the gelatinization and vice versa. It has been demonstrated that the more a starch gelatinizes (because of its low amylose content) the more it can be hydrolyzed by alpha-amylases (starch's digestive enzymes), and the more it tends to be transformed into glucose and the more glycemia tends to rise.

In other words, the less amylose there is in a starch, the higher its glycemic index. In contrast, the higher the proportion of amylose, the lower the amount of gelatinization, the lower the transformation into glucose and the lower the glycemic index.

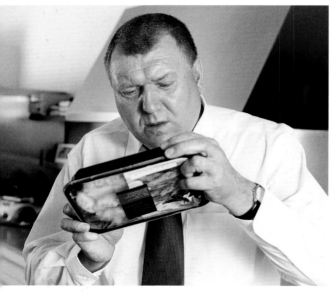

From this we can see why potatoes, with very low amylose content, have high glycemic indexes when cooked in water. We also see why lentils, with high amylose content, have low glycemic index.

Corn is another very important example. Waxy corn has hardly any amylose and has specifically selected by the agrifood industry for the very high viscosity of its starch. For this reason it is commonly used to thicken fruit jellies, and give texture to canned and frozen food. It is called corn starch on labels. Since its glycemic index is very high (very close to 100) its use in industrially prepared food is an important factor and adds to glycemia.

By contrast, an interesting experiment was performed in Australia where an industrial bread manufacturer added a portion of a special corn that has a very high amylose content (>80%) to reduce the glycemic index of a traditional bread. The public, in particular children, who tend to complain about eating whole-wheat bread, apparently welcomed it.

- **The type of technical and heat treatment that the food is subjected to**

Hydration and heat increase a food's glycemic index. Raw carrots, for example, have a glycemic index of 35. When they are boiled their index goes up to 85 because of starch gelatinization.

There are industrial processes that maximize gelatinization. These include manufacture of potato flakes (for instant mashed potatoes) or corn flakes, and also of binders such as modified starches and dextrinized starches. These processes considerably increase glycemic index (85 for corn flakes, 95 for potato flakes, 100 for modified starches). In the same way, exploding a grain of corn to produce pop corn or a grain of rice to make puffed rice increases glycemic index by 15-20% from its starting point.

- **Pastification reduces glycemic index**

There is a natural technique that tends to slow down starch hydration. This is pastification of durum wheat during pasta manufacture. The pasta is extruded through a channel. This heats up the proteins, which means a protective film forms that slows starch gelatinization when they are cooked.

This is mainly valid for spaghetti and some noodles like tagliatelle, that are pastified, i.e. extruded under high pressure, so it is not valid for ravioli or lasagna, nor for fresh pasta that is cut using a pasta roller. These pastas have a much higher glycemic index, even though they are made of the same durum wheat flour.

So from a single kind of flour, we can obtain products whose glycemic indexes are much lower than those of other products (ravioli 70, spaghetti 40).

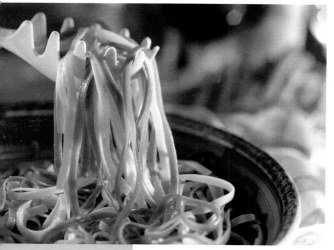

The way the pasta is cooked in a home just prior to being eaten will also affect its final glycemic index. Cooking spaghetti until al dente (5-6 minutes) keeps glycemic index lowest, whereas longer cooking time of 15-20 minutes increases GI because starch gelatinization accelerates.

- **Retrogradation: The Opposite of Gelatinization**

After having being cooked with gelatinization occurring, when starch cools down it changes again. The same thing happens when some foods are dried.

Progressively, the amylose and amylopectin macromolecules reorganize and the gel changes. This is called retrogradation and it is a return to varying degrees to the former molecular structure. Retrogradation increases over time and as temperature drops. Prolonged storage of amylaceous foods at low temperature (5 °C) (e.g. dishes prepared and stored under vacuum) favors retrogradation. In old bread, as humidity migrates to the outside of the bread it favors starch retrogradation. This also happens when bread is toasted.

Even if the retrogradation does not completely reverse gelatinization it does reduce glycemic index. This is why spaghetti (even white spaghetti) cooked al dente then cooled and eaten in a salad will have GI of around 35.

We can also deduce that a bread will not have the same glycemic index when it is eaten freshly cooked (and still warm), a few days old, or toasted. In the same way we can imagine that freezing fresh bread then defrosting it at room temperature might reduce its glycemic index a little.

Another interesting example is that cold green lentils (especially if they have been in the refrigerator for 24 hours) have a lower glycemic index than freshly cooked lentils (between 10 and 15). This happens because the higher the amylose content in the original starch, the more effective the retrogradation. This is also the case for basmati rice, which has a lower glycemic index after having been cooked and cooled than when it is reheated.

It has also been shown that adding lipids to a starch that has been gelatinized slows retrogradation. It is good to know that a retrograded starch that is reheated loses some of its ability to gelatinize. A fraction (about 10%) of the retrograded starch becomes heat-resistant, which points towards reheating a carbohydrate after having been stored in the cold, reducing glycemic index.

Lastly, it is important to mention that native starch (raw and natural) is not only present in raw foods. In some cases it can persist in this form after cooking when the product's water content was locally insufficient to cause gelatinization. This is the case for bread crusts and shortbread-type cookies where the granular

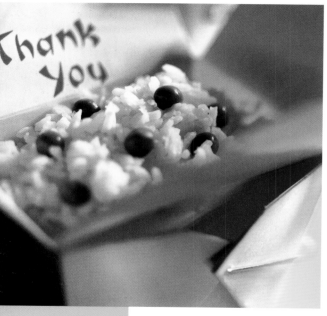

structure persists in part after cooking, reducing their glycemic index compared to starches that were gelatinized (like the inside of the loaf of bread for example). This is also why gentle steaming or cooking 'à l'étouffée', techniques using small amounts of water compared to other methods, causes less gelatinization.

- **Protein and fiber content**

For some carbohydrates, the natural protein content can cause less starch hydrolysis (digestion) and consequently lower glycemic index. This is the case for cereals more than the other families. The phenomenon is particularly clear for pasta. Gluten's presence slows digestive amylases, which limits glucose absorption.

So we see why durum wheat (higher gluten content) has a higher glycemic index than common wheat for bread. Generally speaking though, all high-yield modern wheats have two or three times less gluten that ancient wheats.

Modern cereals are more likely to generate high glycemia when they are eaten refined, which contributes to reducing their gluten content even more, although it is low to start with.

It also seems that a starch's dietary fiber content can constitute a barrier for amylase action and again reduce glucose absorption. Nevertheless, it does seem that it is essentially soluble fibers (found most often in pulses but also in oats) that can play a direct or indirect role in reducing intestinal glucose absorption and reduce the glycemic index of the starch in question.

- **Degree of ripening and aging**

Amylaceous fruits have higher glycemic index the riper they are. This phenomenon is particularly great for bananas, and much less so for apples. A green banana has a quite low glycemic index (about 40). Once it is fully ripe it will be much higher (65) because of its starch transforming as it ripens and becoming more and more resistant. Cooking a green banana has the same effect.

To be as exhaustive as possible, we should note that storing some foods, potatoes in particular, increases GI because of natural starch transformation. Potatoes that have been stores for several months have a higher glycemic index than new potatoes.

- **Acidity**

Studies have shown that acidity reduces a carbohydrate's glycemic index. This is particularly so for bread manufacture. A bread made with standard white flour and yeast will have a GI of 70. But if in place of the yeast the baker uses natural sourdough, the GI will only be 60 or 65. It is the sourdough's acidity that reduces the flour's GI.

In the same way, eating an acidic product during a meal helps to reduce the meal's glycemic balance. This is why the Montignac Method recommends that for example, if you lapse by eating French fries with a high GI (95) in phase II, you should eat them with a salad with an acidic, vinegary dressing. According to Professor J. Brand-Miller, 20 ml of vinegar mixed with 10 ml olive oil would reduce the blood glucose level by 30%.

- **Particle size**

When an amylaceous starch is ground, smaller starch particles make hydrolysis easier, therefore increase glycemic index. This is particularly the case for cereals when they have reduced flour content. Many French health food stores sell a T150 Organic wheat flour whose manufacturer claims a special manufacturing process that is supposedly developed for easier digestion. The process in this case is milling the flour so finely that the glycemic index is as high as a white flour's. The problem is that the vendors sell this flour as "whole grain." For the same reasons, rice flour has a much higher GI that the original rice.

When wheat was ground using stone grinders it was in

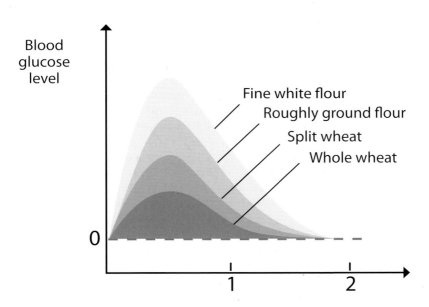

Figure 9: **The larger the particles, the lower the glycemic index**

large particles. Even if it was sifted, a hand-sifting was rough and the resulting flour was rough (partially whole grain flour). White bread at the time had a GI that was about 60-65 which was reasonable.

Ordinary bread was once made with crude, unrefined flour that had all of the wheat grain's original components, which is of course where it gets its "whole grain" name. As the particles were quite large and contained high fiber and protein content and moreover the flour was made using sourdough, the glycemic index was obviously even lower (35-45).

Whole-grain Montignac bread sold online at www.pain-integral-montignac.com and in the "Première Moisson" bakeries in Quebec meets these specifications.

 When the roll mill was invented in 1870, white flour manufacture became common, first in the west, then all over the world. This new technique was obviously considered to be progress, but would lead to a drop in bread's nutritional quality.

Since then, thanks to more and more sophisticated milling equipment, flours are purer and purer, technically speaking. Nutritionally this means: less fiber, less protein and micro-nutrients (vitamins, minerals, essential fatty acids, etc.) and finer and finer particles. This is why foods where this over-refined flour is a major component have ever-increasing glycemic indexes.

Nutrients	Montignac whole grain bread (per 100 g)	White flour (pour 100 g)
Protéin	12 g	8 g
Fat	2,5 g	1 g
Carbohydrate	60 g	74 g
Fiber	14 g	3 g
Water	11,5 g	14 g
Particle size	Large	Fine
Glycemic index	**34** [*]	**70**

Montignac whole-wheat bread

* Calculation performed *in vitro* by an independent approved laboratory.

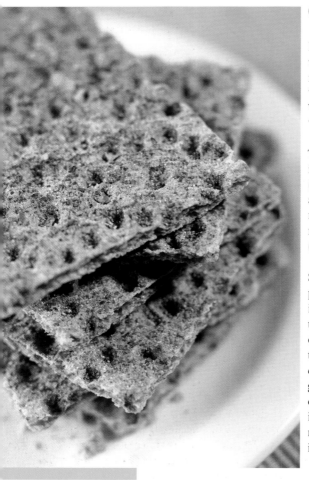

Conclusion

From this we conclude that the variation in carbohydrates nutrition merits close attention. 'Starch' is not a single category. We have to talk about 'starches'.

There are different kinds, first in their molecular structure (amylose/amylopectin ratio) and from the content and nature of the additional nutrients that are also present (protein, fiber).

Starches' physicochemical properties change constantly in the presence of water, temperature variations and over time. Each heat and water treatment, whether industrial or culinary, transforms the food to give it different properties and digestibility. There is a specific intestinal absorption that results in related glycemia and insulin response.

A food's glycemic index is therefore the result of many parameters that we have to account for when selecting our food.

By ignoring the value of these scientific ideas, even though they have been known for more than twenty years now, "traditional nutrition" has let the agri-food industry develop not only problematic botanical varieties, but also and especially, industrial, cooking and storage processes that indirectly raise postprandial glycemia in those who eat modern food, in an alarming way.

We know today that hyperinsulinism is the final stage in this problematic metabolism, and that it causes the high levels of obesity, diabetes and much cardiovascular disease. From now on we can measure the imprudence of official nutritional recommendations for the public.

We are told to eat 50-55% carbohydrates in our daily diet without mention of which types of carbohydrates they should be. Even worse, if the type were mentioned, it still refers to the classification of sugars as fast and slow, which we know is totally wrong.

As Professor Walter Willet from Harvard Medical School says, these recommendations are never accompanied by explanations about treatment (cooking, storage) of these carbohydrates in view of their glycemic index.

Although the official advice is to eat complex carbohydrates this does not have much effect given current nutritional understanding. As scientists F. Bornet and Professor G. Slama have said, not only are complex carbohydrates *not interchangeable,* as we thought was the case for a long time, but we have to understand that *some starches or amylaceous foods, although they are complex, are more hyperglycemiant than simple sugars.* For example fried potatoes (GI 95) are more hyperglycemiant than sugar (GI 70).

After having been the first nutritionist in the world to propose using glycemic index for weight loss, I have endeavored to show for more than twenty years in all of my publications, how the drift in eating habits over the last fifty years has caused increased worldwide obesity.

By passing from eating habits that caused little glycemia (with a diet composed mainly of carbohydrates with low and very low glycemic index) which was how our ancestors eat, to eating habits that are hyperglycemiant (composed largely of high and very high glycemic index carbohydrates), a higher proportion of people have developed metabolic diseases, and especially hyperinsulinism, which is the determining factor for weight gain and diabetes.

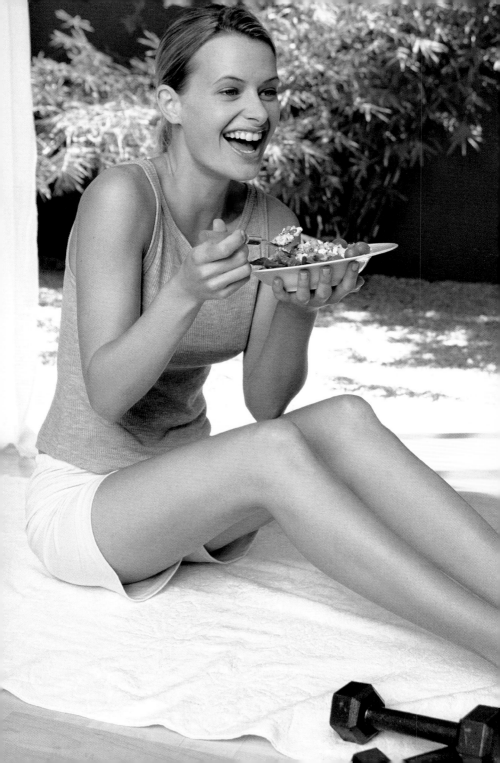

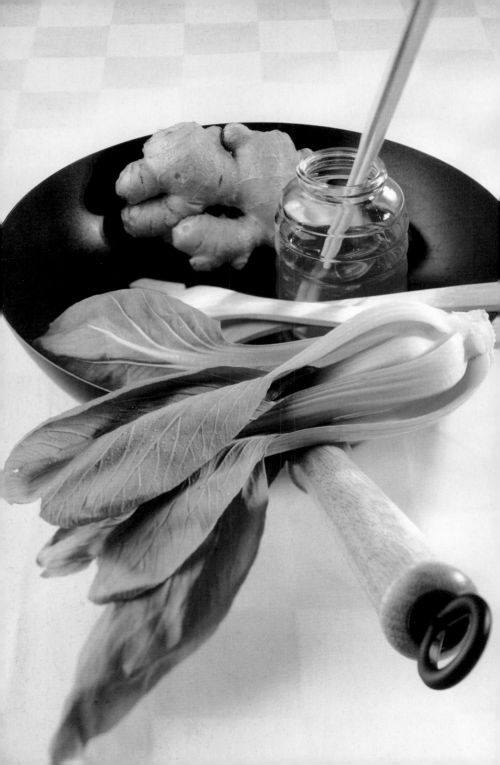

Clarifications regarding Glycemic Indexes

Glycemic Index is an Average Value

We must remember that a food's glycemic index (GI) is an average value. First of all it is the average of the individual effects seen on a group of people.

Then it is also an average of calculations made for different foods that fall within the same category. For a cereal like wheat, for example, varieties' specific protein and fiber contents can lead to slightly different numbers.

The tables indicate the average values, and we do sometimes give a range. For example, we say that the GI of white flour is 69 (±6) which means that the flours tested gave a maximum value of 75 and a minimum of 65.

Therefore a food's glycemic index (GI) is approximate by definition. It is an indicative value.

A food's GI is more an indication than an exact value. This is why in the Montignac Method the GI given are compared to averages that have been rounded to the closest category.

This approach is much simpler and does not detract from its worth

Watch out for GI Classifications! They are wrong most of the time.

The glycemic index classification that most authors give is generally incorrect. GI are in principal classified in three categories: High, medium and low

Most authors consider:

- that GI below 55 are **low**;
- that GI between 55 and 69 are **medium**;
- that GI above 70 are **high**;

But this grouping does not correspond to any physiological reality. It is just politically correct as it has been constructed arbitrarily with the food industry so that most of existing products do not fall into the high GI category.

However, it was also established to appease traditional nutritionists whose nutritional recommendations (potatoes, cereals, etc.) would be found in the high GI column (so would be suspect) if we had remained objective. This is why we have to be careful of all the tables that we find in books and on the internet, that have been established from incorrect principles.

Since their authors have little or no experience in GI, they simply copied what had been said before by a few authorities on the matter, and authorities who were more consensual and pro-business than scientific.

The right classification

The classification that best respects the reality of digestive physiology is as follows:

- Low GI are less than or equal to 35
- Average GI are between 35 and 50
- High GI are above 50.

This classification could also be refined as follows:

- Low GI are below 50, and very low GI are below 35
- High GI are above 50.

Watch out for the contradictory information in some tables!

Since glycemic index has been discovered, two methods of calculation have been proposed to establish tables.

Some scientists built their tables giving white bread a value of 100, and most gave glucose a value of 100.

The first group was obviously wrong in having taken a naturally variable value as a basis for calculation (the G of white bread varies according to the origin of the wheat, the milling and the flour and the fermentation and cooking process).

Glucose is a better reference because it always causes the same physiological reaction, which is the intestinal absorption of 100% of the pure carbohydrate it contains.

Unfortunately, GI tables coming from different methods of calculation are circulating and cohabiting in nature (on the Internet in particular) without stating their origin. An even worse situation though, is that we often find (in books and on the Internet) compilations of tables of various origins whose values do not correspond. So watch out!

The glycemic index table that we give in this book is not exhaustive, nor definitive. It was established from various values determined over many studies from which we used the averages.

Readers of Montignac Method books are sometimes surprised when they see that the values are different here than in other books. They could be surprised, for example in seeing that sugar-free whole grain cereals have a GI of 45 where they are still listed as having a GI of 40 in most books.

The reason is simple: For a long time we had hardly any studies to refer to. Everything published since has led to new averages.

This is why for many foods GI are higher or lower. Our intention is to update the values indicated the table for each new issue as new information becomes available.

Glycemic Load

Glycemia, as we have seen, is the blood glucose level and the result of two factors: A food's glycemic index and also the amount of pure carbohydrate that it contains.

But if you eat 100g cooked carrots whose GI is high (85), the glycemia cause will paradoxically be low for the good reason that carrot have low carbohydrate content (5%).

If you eat a very-low GI carbohydrate like fructose (GI = 20) but you eat a lot of it (100 g for example) the glycemia will be paradoxically much higher, in spite of the low GI, because the carbohydrate content is at a maximum (100 g per 100 g).

Research scientists at Harvard University have turned this into an equation by creating a new concept called glycemic load. The glycemic load (GL) is found by multiplying a food's glycemic index (GI) by its carbohydrate content (content in grams in a serving) and dividing the result by 100:

GL = (GI x pure carbohydrate content for 100 g)/100

EXAMPLE:

Carrots: 85 x 5/100 = **4.25** GL

Fructose: 20 x 100/100 = **20** GL

The value of GL is that it shows that some carbohydrates (such as fructose) can cause high glycemia in spite of low GI and that other high GI

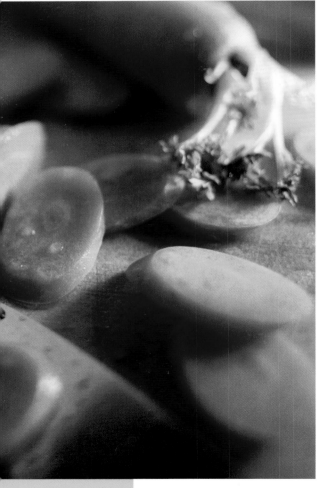

carbohydrates (such as coked carrots) only have slight effect on glycemia because of their low GI. The parameter is pure carbohydrate content.

Some people believed that GL would knock GI off its pedestal because it was much more precise, but even though it is technically interesting, it has two major drawbacks in our opinion:

• It is of limited value because apart from a few extreme products like those used in the examples, it does not offer anything extra in selections of common foods.

• It is complicated!

Many people already find glycemic index difficult to understand. Therefore it seems useless to further complicate the situation with another concept that does not add much to the practical details.

This is why I am content with listing a few exceptions to carbohydrate indexes that can be summarized very briefly as follows:

• There are some high GI carbohydrates that can still be eaten as if they had low GI because they contain very little pure carbohydrate.

Examples include cooked carrots, and melons and watermelons.

• There are some low GI carbohydrates whose quantity should be restricted. Fructose is the main item in this category, since it contains 100% pure carbohydrate.

This is why in the Montignac Method I recommend that no more than 30g fructose be eaten per day.

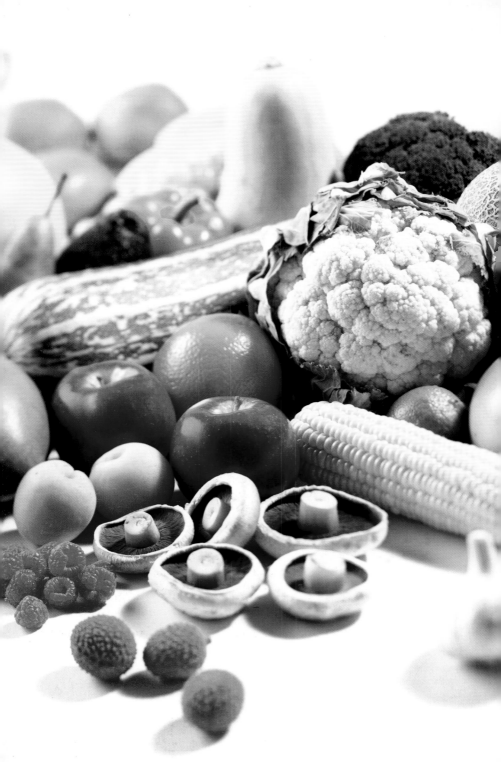

GI index:
classification tables

You'll find two GI classification tables on the following pages.

The first lists the foods in alphabetical order, the second by glycemic index.

We are going to use the following legend:
* Even if they have a high GI, these foods have a very low carbohydrate content (around 5%). Thus eating them in a normal quantity should have a negligible affect on glycemia.

** There is practically no difference in GI between whole dairy products and fat-free dairy products. It is important to remember that even if dairy products have a low GI, their insulin index is high.

*** These foods do not contain carbohydrate and have a GI of 0.

GI table: Alphabetical classification

A

Acerola	20
Apple (compote)	35
Apple (fresh)	30
Apple juice (sugar-free)	40
Dried apples	35
Agave (syrup)	15
Alcohol	0
All Bran™	50
Almonds	15
Almond milk	30
Blanched almond puree (without sugar)	35
Unrefined almond puree (without sugar)	25
Amaranth	35
Puffed amaranth	70
Apricots (canned, in syrup)	60
Apricots (fresh)	30
Dried apricots	35
Arrow-root	85
Artichokes	20
Jerusalem artichokes	50
Asparagus	15
Avocado	10

B

Bagels	70
Baguette, white bread (T)	70
Bamboo shoots	20
Bananas (unripened)	45
Bananas (ripe)	60
Adzuki beans	35
Borlotti beans	35
Green beans, French beans, snow peas	15
White beans, cannellini beans	35
Mung beans (soy)	25
Black beans	35
Kidney beans	35
Kidney beans (canned)	40
Green beans	30
Beets (raw)	30
Beets (cooked)*	65
Beer*	110

GI table: Alphabetical classification

Beef*** (steak, filet, rib steak, etc.)	0
Bilberries	25
Blackberries	25
Blueberries	25
Bread without gluten (rice flour + potato starch)	90
Brown bread (sourdough)	65
Essene bread (made from sprouts)	35
Kamut bread	45
Matzo bread (white flour)	70
Matzo bread (unrefined flour)	40
100% whole-wheat pure sourdough bread	40
Quinoa bread (around % quinoa)	50
Rice bread	70
Rye bread (around % rye)	65
Standard unrefined bread	65
Standard whole-wheat bread	45
Toasted bread, unrefined flour without sugar	45
Very white bread, sandwich bread (like Harry's®)	85
Whole grain rye bread	65
Montignac® real whole-wheat bread	34
Hamburger bun	85
Bulgur (wheat, cooked)	55
Bulgur (wheat)	45
Unrefined bulgur (wheat, cooked)	45
Bran (wheat, oat, etc.)	15
Brioches	70
Broccoli	15
Broad beans (cooked)	80
Broad beans (raw)	40
Breadfruit	65
Hulled barley	25
Pearl barley	60
Buckwheat (whole grain: flour or bread)	40
C	
Cabbage	15
Capellini	45
Carob powder	15
Carrots (raw)	30
Carrots (cooked)*	85
Cassoulet	35
Cashews	15

GI table: Alphabetical classification

Cauliflower	15
Celery	15
Celeriac (raw; rémoulade)	35
Celeriac (cooked)*	85
Cereal energy bar (sugar-free)	50
Champignons	15
Swiss chard	15
Chayote, christophene (puree)	50
Cheeses (gruyere, camembert, Swiss, edam, feta, goat cheese, gouda, parmesan)***/**	0
Cherries	25
Chestnuts	60
Chicory (drink)	40
Chicory syrup	55
Chips	70
Cold cuts (sausages, salami, coppa, etc.) ham (white, ham, prosciutto, smoked, etc.)***	0
Cocoa powder (with sugar)	60
Cocoa powder (sugar-free)	20
Coffee, tea and herb tea***	0
Coconuts	35
Coconut milk	40
Chocolate bar (sugar-free Montignac® type)	35
Dark chocolate (> 70% cocoa)	25
Dark chocolate (> 85% cocoa)	20
Dry cider	40
Cointreau®	60
Coke, carbonated soft drinks, sodas (like Coca-Cola®)	70
Cookies	55
Cookies (whole-wheat, sugar-free)	50
Corn Flakes	85
Corn mush	70
Indian corn	35
Corn syrup	115
Corn in kernels	65
Cornstarch	85
Cornichon	15
Couscous, semolina	65
Unrefined couscous, semolina	50
Whole grain couscous, semolina	45
cranberries	45

GI table: Alphabetical classification

cranberry juice (sugar-free)	50
Crème fraîche***/**	0
Croissant	70
Cucumber	15
Red current	25
Black current	15
D	
Dates	70
Doughnuts	75
E	
Endive, chicory	15
Eggplant	20
Eggs***	0
F	
Falafel (broad beans)	40
Falafel (chick peas)	35
Fennel	15
Fig; prickly pair (fresh)	30
Dried figs	35
Flageolet beans	25
Flour (whole-wheat)	45
Flour (Ebly®)	45
Corn flour	70
Chestnut flour	65
Chick pea flour	35
Spelt flour (whole grain)	45
Kamut flour (whole grain)	45
Quinoa flour	40
Rice flour	95
Soy flour	25
Unrefined flour (wheat)	60
Wheatmeal flour (wheat)	65
White wheat flour	85
Foie gras	15
French fries	95
Fresh fruit juice sugar-free	40
Fromage blanc** undrained	30
Montignac® fructose	20
G	
Garlic	30
Ginger	15

GI table: Alphabetical classification

Glucose	100
Glucose syrup	100
Gnocchi	70
Goose fat, vegetable fat, margarine***	0
Gooseberry	25
Grape (fresh)	45
Grapefruit (fresh)	30
Grapefruit juice (sugar-free)	45
Grape juice (sugar-free)	65
Sugary refined grains	70
Whole grains (without sugar)	45
H	
Hazelnuts	15
Whole hazelnut puree (sugar-free)	25
Heart of palm	20
Honey	60
Hummus	25
I	
Ice cream (with fructose)	35
Traditional ice cream (with sugar)	60
J	
Jam (marmalade) without sugar (concentrated grape juice)	45
Montignac® sugar-free jam (marmalade)	20
Standard jam (with sugar)	60/65
K	
Whole grain kamut	40
Ketchup	55
Kiwi*	45
L	
Lactose	40
Lasagna (hard wheat)	55
Lasagna (soft wheat)	75
Leeks	15
Lemon	20
Lemon juice (sugar-free)	15
Brown lentils	30
Yellow lentils	30
Green lentils	25
Linseed, sesame, poppy (seeds)	35
Litchi (fresh)	50
Lupine	15

GI table: Alphabetical classification

M

Macaroni (hard wheat)	50
Mango (fresh)	45
Mango juice (sugar-free)	55
Maple syrup	65
Marie-Brizard®	60
Mars®, Snickers®, Nuts®, etc.	65
Mayonnaise (natural: egg, oil and mustard)	0
Mayonnaise (industrial, with sugar)	60
Meats (beef, pork, poultry, lamb, mutton, rabbit, sausages, blood sausage, dried beef, etc.)***	0
Melon*	60
Medlar	55
Milk** (skim or not)	30
Fresh/powdered milk**	30
Millet, sorghum	70
Molasses	70
Muesli (with sugar, honey, etc.)	65
Muesli (without sugar)	50
Mustard	35
Mustard (with sugar added)	55

N

Nectarines (white or yellow; fresh fruit)	35
Nutella®	55

O

Oats	40
Oatmeal	60
Oatmeal (raw)	40
Oat milk (raw)	30
Oils (Olive, sunflower, etc)***	0
Olives	15
Onions	15
Oranges (fresh)	35
Orange juice (sugar-free)	45
Ovaltine®	60

P

Pain au chocolat	65
Pain au lait	60
Papaya (fresh)	55
Passion fruit, purple granadilla	30
Pasta (soft wheat)	70

GI table: Alphabetical classification

Pasta/Ravioli	65
Unrefined pasta (whole-wheat)	50
Whole-wheat pasta (al dente)	40
Peaches (canned, in syrup)	55
Peaches (fresh)	35
Peanuts	15
Peanut butter (without sugar added)	40
Peanut puree (sugar-free)	25
Pears (fresh)	30
Peas (canned)	45
Peas (fresh)	35
Split peas	25
Chick peas (canned)	35
Pepino, melon pear	40
Hot pepper	15
Bell peppers	15
Pernod-Ricard®	45
Persimmon	50
Pesto	15
Physalis	15
Pineapple (canned)	65
Pineapple (fresh)	45
Pineapple juice (sugar-free)	50
Pine nut	15
Pineau®	45
Pistachio	15
Standard pizza (white flour)	60
Plantains (raw)	45
Plantains (cooked)	70
Plums (fresh)	30
Polenta, corn meal	70
Potatoes cooked in skin (water/steam)	65
Potato starch	95
Poultry (chicken, turkey, etc.)***	0
Sweet potatoes	50
Mashed potato mix (instant)	90
Mashed potato	80
Baked potatoes	95
Boiled, peeled potatoes	70
Pop corn (without sugar)	85
Porto®	45

GI table: Alphabetical classification

Pumpkin*	75
Prunes	35
Standard pumpernickel	45
Montignac® pumpernickel	40
Pomegranate (fresh)	35
Pumpkin seeds	25
Q	
Quinoa	35
Quince (fresh)	35
Quince jelly (sugar-free)	40
Quince jelly (with sugar)	65
R	
Radish	15
Raisins	65
Raspberries (fresh)	25
Ratatouille	20
Ravioli (hard wheat)	55
Ravioli (soft wheat)	70
Rhubarb	15
Risotto	70
Camargue rice (white)	60
Fragrant rice (jasmine, etc.)	60
Glutinous rice	90
Instant/parboiled rice (precooked)	85
Long grain rice (white)	60
Long grain basmati rice	50
Montignac® long grain unrefined basmati rice	40
Puffed rice, rice cakes	85
Red rice	55
Rice noodles	30
Rice cake	85
Rice milk	85
Rice with milk (with sugar)	75
Standard white rice	70
Unrefined basmati rice	45
Unrefined brown rice	50
Wild rice	35
Rutabaga	70
Rye (whole grain; flour or bread)	45
S	
Salad (lettuce, escarole, curly endive, lamb's lettuce, etc.)	15

GI table: Alphabetical classification

Salsify	30
Sauerkraut	15
Sea food*** (shrimp, mussels, oysters, etc.)	0
Seed sprouts	15
Semolina	50
Shallot	15
Shellfish (lobster, crab, spiny lobster, etc.)	5
Sherbet (without sugar)	40
Sherbet (with sugar)	65
Shortbread (flour, butter and sugar)	55
Shortbread (whole-wheat, sugar-free)	40
Montignac® whole-wheat shortbread	35
Soursop, sugar apple	35
Spaghetti al dente (cooked 5 min)	40
Well-cooked white spaghetti	55
Low GI Montignac® spaghetti 10	10
Special K® (Kellogg's®)	75
Spelt	40
Spelt (whole grain flour)	45
Spelt (refined flour)	65
Spelt (whole grain bread)	45
Spices (pepper, parsley, basil, caraway, cinnamon, vanilla, etc.)	5
Spinach	15
Sprouts (wheat, soy, etc.)	15
Brussels sprouts	15
Squashes (various)*	75
Soja cuisine	20
Sorrel	15
Soy (seeds/beans)	15
Soy milk	30
Soy sauce (sugar-free, no sweeteners)	15
Soybean noodles	30
Modified starches	100
Strawberries (fresh)	25
White sugar (saccharose)	70
Brown sugar	70
Dried sugarcane juice	65
Sunflower (seeds)	35
Surimi	50
Sushi	55

GI table: Alphabetical classification

T

Tacos	70
Tagliatelle (well-cooked)	55
Tahini	40
Tamari (sugar-free, no sweeteners)	15
Tamarind (sweet)	65
Tangerines	30
Tapioca	85
Tempeh	15
Tofu (soy)	15
Tomatoes	30
Tomato sauce (with sugar)	45
Tomato sauce (without sugar)	35
Tomato juice	35
Dried tomatoes	35
Turnip (raw)	30
Turnip (cooked)*	85
Turnips*	85

V

Hard wheat vermicelli	40
Balsamic vinegar	5

W

Waffle with sugar	75
Wasa fiber ™ (24%)	35
Wasa light ™	50
Watermelon*	75
Cooked wine (Martini®, etc.)	40
Liquorous wine	30
Red wine, white wine, champagne*** dry sparkling wine	0
Wheat syrup, rice syrup	100

Y

Yam	65
Yeast	35
Brewer's yeast	35
Yogurt (plain)	30
Soy milk yogurt (flavored)	35
Soy milk yogurt (plain)	20

Z

Zucchini	15
Zwieback	70

GI table: Classification by GI

GI>50

Corn syrup	115
Beer*	110
Modified starches	100
Glucose	100
Wheat syrup, rice syrup	100
Glucose syrup	100
Rice flour	95
Potato starch	95
Baked potatoes	95
French fries	95
Bread without gluten (rice flour + potato starch)	90
Mashed potato mix (instant)	90
Glutinous rice	90
Arrow-root	85
Carrots (cooked)*	85
Celeriac (cooked)*	85
Corn Flakes	85
White wheat flour T45	85
Rice cake	85
Rice milk	85
Cornstarch	85
Turnip (cooked)*	85
Hamburger bun	85
Very white bread, sandwich bread (like Harry's®)	85
Turnips*	85
Pop corn (without sugar)	85
Instant/parboiled rice (precooked)	85
Puffed rice, rice cakes	85
Tapioca	85
Cooked broad beans	80
Mashed potato	80
Squashes (various)*	75
Doughnuts	75
Waffle with sugar	75
Lasagna (soft wheat)	75
Watermelon*	75
Pumpkin*	75
Rice with milk (with sugar)	75
Special K® (Kellogg's®)	75

GI table: Classification by GI

Puffed amaranth	**70**
Bagels	**70**
Baguette, white bread (T55)	**70**
Plantains (cooked)	**70**
Zwieback	**70**
Corn mush	**70**
Brioches	**70**
Sugary refined grains	**70**
Chips	**70**
Coke, carbonated soft drinks, sodas (like Coca-Cola®)	**70**
Croissant	**70**
Dates	**70**
Corn flour	**70**
Gnocchi	**70**
Molasses	**70**
Millet, sorghum	**70**
Pasta (soft wheat)	**70**
Matzo bread (white flour)	**70**
Rice bread	**70**
Polenta, corn meal	**70**
Boiled, peeled potatoes	**70**
Ravioli (soft wheat)	**70**
Risotto	**70**
Standard white rice	**70**
Rutabaga	**70**
White sugar (saccharose)	**70**
Brown sugar	**70**
Tacos	**70**
Pineapple (canned)	**65**
Beets (cooked)*	**65**
Standard jam with sugar	**65**
Standard jam with sugar	**60/65**
Couscous, semolina	**65**
Spelt (refined flour)	**65**
Chestnut flour	**65**
Wheatmeal flour (wheat)	**65**
Breadfruit	**65**
Quince jelly (with sugar)	**65**
Yam	**65**
Dried sugarcane juice	**65**
Grape juice (sugar-free)	**65**

GI table: Classification by GI

Corn in kernels	65
Mars®, Snickers®, Nuts®, etc.	65
Muesli (with sugar, honey, etc.)	65
Pasta/Ravioli	65
Pain au chocolat	65
Rye bread (around 30% rye)	65
Brown bread (sourdough)	65
Standard unrefined bread	65
Whole grain rye bread	65
Potatoes cooked in skin (water/steam)	65
Raisins	65
Maple syrup	65
Sherbet (with sugar)	65
Tamarind (sweet)	65
Apricots (canned, in syrup)	60
Bananas (ripe)	60
Chestnuts	60
Cointreau®	60
Traditional ice cream (with sugar)	60
Unrefined flour (wheat)	60
Marie-Brizard®	60
Mayonnaise (industrial, with sugar)	60
Melon*	60
Honey	60
Pearl barley	60
Ovaltine®	60
Pain au lait	60
Standard pizza (white flour)	60
Oatmeal	60
Cocoa powder (with sugar)	60
Ravioli (hard wheat)	60
Camargue rice (white)	60
Long grain rice (white)	60
Fragrant rice (jasmine, etc.)	60
Semolina	60
Cookies	55
Bulgur (wheat, cooked)	55
Mango juice (sugar-free)	55
Ketchup	55
Lasagna (hard wheat)	55
Cassava (bitter)	55

GI table: Classification by GI

Cassava (sweet)	55
Mustard (with sugar added)	55
Medlar	55
Nutella®	55
Papaya (fresh)	55
Peaches (canned, in syrup)	55
Red rice	55
Chicory syrup	55
Well-cooked white spaghetti	55
Sushi	55
Tagliatelle (well-cooked)	55
GI<50	
All Bran™	50
Cereal energy bar (sugar-free)	50
Cookies (whole-wheat, sugar-free)	50
Chayote, christophene (puree)	50
Unrefined couscous, semolina	50
Red current/cranberry juice (sugar-free)	50
Pineapple juice (sugar-free)	50
Persimmon	50
Litchi (fresh)	50
Macaroni (hard wheat)	50
Muesli (without sugar)	50
Quinoa bread (around 65% quinoa)	50
Sweet potatoes	50
Unrefined pasta (whole-wheat)	50
Long grain basmati rice	50
Unrefined brown rice	50
Surimi	50
Jerusalem artichokes	50
Wasa light ™	50
Red currents, cranberries	45
Pineapple (fresh)	45
Bananas (unripened)	45
Plantains (raw)	45
Flour (whole-wheat)	45
Flour (Ebly®)	45
Unrefined bulgur (wheat, cooked)	45
Capellini	45

GI table: Classification by GI

Whole grains (without sugar)	45
Jam (marmalade) without sugar (concentrated grape juice)	45
Whole grain couscous, semolina	45
Spelt (whole grain flour)	45
Spelt (whole grain bread)	45
Spelt flour (whole grain)	45
Kamut flour (whole grain)	45
Orange juice (sugar-free)	45
Grapefruit juice (sugar-free)	45
Kiwi*	45
Mango (fresh)	45
Kamut bread	45
Toasted bread, unrefined flour without sugar	45
Standard whole-wheat bread	45
Pernod-Ricard®	45
Peas (canned)	45
Bulgur (wheat)	45
Pineau®	45
Porto®	45
Standard pumpernickel	45
Grape (fresh)	45
Unrefined basmati rice	45
Tomato sauce (with sugar)	45
Rye (whole grain; flour or bread)	40
Oats	40
Peanut butter (without sugar added)	40
Chicory (drink)	40
Dry cider	40
Falafel (broad beans)	40
Quinoa flour	40
spelt	40
Broad beans (raw)	40
Dried figs	40
Oatmeal (raw)	40
Quince jelly (sugar-free)	40
Kidney beans (canned)	40
Fresh fruit juice sugar-free	40
Apple juice (sugar-free)	40
Whole grain kamut	40
Lactose	40

GI table: Classification by GI

Coconut milk	40
100% whole-wheat pure sourdough bread	40
Matzo bread (unrefined flour)	40
Whole-wheat pasta (al dente)	40
Pepino, melon pear	40
Montignac® pumpernickel	40
Tahini	40
Montignac® long grain unrefined basmati rice	40
Shortbread (whole-wheat, sugar-free)	40
Buckwheat (whole grain: flour or bread)	40
Sherbet (without sugar)	40
Spaghetti al dente (cooked 5 min)	40
Hard wheat vermicelli	40
Cooked wines (Martini®, etc.)	40

GI<35

Dried apricots	35
Amaranth	35
Soursop, sugar apple	35
Chocolate bar (sugar-free Montignac® type)	35
Nectarines (white or yellow; fresh fruit)	35
Cassoulet	35
Celeriac (raw; rémoulade)	35
Quince (fresh)	35
Ice cream (with fructose)	35
Falafel (chick peas)	35
Chick pea flour	35
Dried figs	35
Pomegranate (fresh)	35
Adzuki beans	35
Borlotti beans	35
Black beans	35
Kidney beans	35
Tomato juice	35
Yeast	35
Brewer's yeast	35
Linseed, sesame, poppy (seeds)	35
Indian corn	35
Mustard	35
Coconuts	35

GI table: Classification by GI

Oranges (fresh)	35
Essene bread (made from sprouts)	35
Peaches (fresh)	35
Peas (fresh)	35
Chick peas (canned)	35
Apple (compote)	35
Dried apples	35
Prunes	35
Blanched almond puree (without sugar)	35
Quinoa	35
Wild rice	35
Montignac® whole-wheat shortbread	35
Tomato sauce (without sugar)	35
Dried tomatoes	35
Sunflower (seeds)	35
Wasa fiber ™ (24%)	35
Soy milk yogurt (flavored)	35
Montignac® real whole-wheat bread	34
Apricots (fresh)	30
Garlic	30
Beets (raw)	30
Carrots (raw)	30
Fig, prickly pair (fresh)	30
Fromage blanc** undrained	30
Passion fruit, purple granadilla	30
Green beans	30
Almond milk	30
Oat milk (raw)	30
Soy milk	30
Fresh/powdered milk**	30
Milk** (skim or not)	30
Brown lentils	30
Yellow lentils	30
Tangerines	30
Turnip (raw)	30
Grapefruit (fresh)	30
Pears (fresh)	30
Apple (fresh)	30
Plums (fresh)	30
Salsify	30
Tomatoes	30

GI table: Classification by GI

Soybean noodles	30
Rice noodles	30
Liquorous wine	30
Yogurt (plain)	30
Bilberries, blueberries	25
Cherries	25
Dark chocolate (> 70% cocoa)	25
Soy flour	25
Flageolet beans	25
Strawberries (fresh)	25
Raspberries (fresh)	25
Pumpkin seeds	25
Red current	25
Gooseberry	25
Mung beans (soy)	25
Hummus	25
Green lentils	25
Blackberries	25
Blueberries, bilberry	25
Hulled barley	25
Split peas	25
Unrefined almond puree (without sugar)	25
Peanut puree (sugar-free)	25
Whole hazelnut puree (sugar-free)	25
Artichokes	20
Eggplant	20
Cocoa powder (sugar-free)	20
Acerola	20
Dark chocolate (> 85% cocoa)	20
Lemon	20
Heart of palm	20
Montignac® sugar-free jam (marmalade)	20
Montignac® fructose	20
Bamboo shoots	20
Ratatouille	20
Soja cuisine	20
Soy milk yogurt (plain)	20
Agave (syrup)	15
Almonds	15
Asparagus	15
Swiss chard	15

GI table: Classification by GI

Broccoli	15
Cashews, peanuts	15
Black currents	15
Celery	15
Sprouts (wheat, soy, etc.)	15
Champignons	15
Sauerkraut	15
Cauliflower	15
Cabbage	15
Brussels sprouts	15
Cucumber	15
Cornichon	15
Zucchini	15
Shallot	15
Endive, chicory	15
Spinach	15
Fennel	15
Foie gras	15
Ginger	15
Seed sprouts	15
Black current	15
Green beans, French beans, snow peas	15
Lemon juice (sugar-free)	15
Lupine	15
Hazelnuts	15
Cashews	15
Onions	15
Olives	15
Sorrel	15
Pesto	15
Physalis	15
Pine nut	15
Hot pepper	15
Pistachio	15
Leeks	15

GI table: Classification by GI

Bell peppers	15
Carob powder	15
Radish	15
Rhubarb	15
Salad (lettuce, escarole, curly endive, lamb's lettuce, etc.)	15
Soy sauce (sugar-free, no sweeteners)	15
Tamari (sugar-free, no sweeteners)	15
Soy (seeds/beans)	15
Bran (wheat, oat, etc.)	15
Tempeh	15
Tofu (soy)	15
Avocado	10
Low GI Montignac® spaghetti	10
Shellfish (lobster, crab, spiny lobster, etc.)	5
Spices (pepper, parsley, basil, caraway, cinnamon, vanilla, etc.)	5
Balsamic vinegar	5
GI>0	
Alcohol	0
Beef*** (steak, filet, rib steak, etc.)	0
Coffee, tea and herb tea***	0
Cold cuts (sausages, salami, coppa, etc.) ham (white, ham, prosciutto, smoked, etc.)***	0
Crème fraîche***/**	0
Cheeses (gruyere, camembert, Swiss, edam, feta, goat cheese, gouda, parmesan)***/**	0
Sea food*** (shrimp, mussels, oysters, etc.)	0
Goose fat, vegetable fat, margarine***	0
Oils (Olive, sunflower, etc)***	0
Mayonnaise (natural: egg, oil and mustard)	0
Eggs***	0
Meats (beef, pork, poultry, veal, lamb, rabbit, etc.)***	0
Red wine, white wine, champagne*** dry sparkling wine	0
Poultry (chicken, turkey, etc.)***	0

In our collection Alpen éditions:

-The Omega-3 Answer

-Living with a Hyperactive Child

-All About the Prostate

-The French Paradox

-The XXL Syndrome

with Michel Montignac:

-Eat Yourself Slim

-The Montignac Diet Cookbook

-The French GI Diet

-Glycemic Index Diet

www.alpen.mc